INTUITIVE DIETING AND WEIGHT LOSS

Beyond the Scale: Embracing Your Body's Wisdom for Effortless Weight Management through Intuitive Dieting

By

Daniel D. Belser

TABLE OF CONTENTS

INTRODUCTION

In a society where strict diet regimens and fast fixes for weight loss are frequently the norm, the paradigm of intuitive dieting stands out as a source of sustainability and balance. Developing a harmonious relationship with one's body, food, and general well-being is encouraged by intuitive dieting, which is more than just a way to lose weight.

The core principle of intuitive dieting is to learn to listen to your body's inherent good judgment. This method helps people to re-establish a connection with their internal cues—listening to hunger, acknowledging fullness, and making thoughtful eating choices—instead of depending on external regulations or meal patterns. It's about regaining the enjoyment of eating and providing your body with the nourishment that feels good for you.

In contrast to traditional weight loss techniques, which frequently emphasize self-deprivation and self-control, intuitive dieting places more emphasis on empowerment and self-awareness. Adopting the tenets of intuitive eating teaches people to trust their bodies and make decisions based on their emotional and physical needs rather than what other people think they should. This paradigm change promotes a healthy relationship with food and sustainable weight loss.

Join us as we explore the transforming potential of self-awareness, mindful practices, and practical ideas as we tackle intuitive dieting and weight loss. This is an invitation to engage on a journey of self-discovery, where health and well-being are attainable and associated with a life lived in harmony with your body. It's more than just a trip to a trimmer physique. Explore the science and practice of intuitive dieting with us as we adopt a comprehensive strategy for living a longer, healthier life.

CHAPTER ONE

OVERVIEW OF INTUITIVE DIETING, AND THE IMPORTANCE OF A MINDFUL APPROACH

1.1 Synopsis of Intuitive Nutrition

Unlike conventional weight loss techniques, intuitive dieting emphasizes a more comprehensive and individualized approach to reaching and maintaining a healthy weight. Fundamentally, intuitive dieting is predicated on the idea that people have an intrinsic capacity to direct their eating behaviors in response to internal cues like hunger, fullness, and contentment.

Basis of Intuitive Dieting: Paying Attention to Your Body Regaining a sense of connection with one's body and learning to recognize hunger and fullness cues are two benefits of intuitive dieting. One can make wise and nourishing decisions by closely observing these indications.

Mindful Eating: Mindful eating is a key component of intuitive dieting. This is living in the moment while eating, appreciating every taste, and encouraging a greater awareness of the sensory aspects of food.

Freedom from Strict Rules: Intuitive dieting encourages a sense of freedom in contrast to traditional diets that impose strict guidelines and calorie limits. It encourages people to choose their foods according to their dietary requirements and tastes.

Awareness of Emotions: The concept of intuitive dieting acknowledges the impact of emotions on eating patterns. It helps people develop healthy relationships by encouraging them to investigate the link between feelings and eating decisions.

Rejecting the Diet Mentality: This strategy aims to help people adopt a longer-term, more sustainable mindset in place of the restrictive dieting cycle. It disproves the idea of "good" and "bad" foods and advocates for a diverse, inclusive, and balanced diet.

Enhanced Welfare: Beyond the scale, intuitive dieting seeks to improve overall health. People who cultivate a pleasant relationship with food frequently are more energized, having better digestion, and emotional health.

Sustainable Lifestyle: Intuitive dieting provides a sustainable lifestyle, as contrast to quick-fix diets, which are frequently difficult to stick to. Because it can be customized to fit certain tastes and situations, it is a workable long-term solution.

1.2 Importance of a Mindful Approach

The value of taking a deliberate approach in the context of intuitive dieting cannot be emphasized. The foundation of this all-encompassing approach is mindfulness, which goes beyond the simple act of eating to promote a deep bond between the body and the mind. When people integrate mindfulness into their eating practices, they go on a transformative journey that impacts their mental, emotional, and spiritual well-being in addition to their weight reduction.

Developing Awareness of the Present Moment: Savoring the Experience Eating mindfully entails giving your complete attention to the flavors, textures, and scents of your food. This increased consciousness makes eating more significant and creates a stronger bond with the food we eat.

Getting Rid of Automatic Patterns: By breaking these tendencies, mindfulness enables people to choose consciously instead of giving in to emotional or mindless eating.

Identifying Hunger and Fullness: People who adopt a mindful approach are better able to separate authentic hunger from other drives. One can better respond to the body's requirements by being aware of internal signs, such as energy levels and stomach sensations.

Avoiding Overeating: Eating mindfully encourages a more acute sense of fullness, which aids in preventing overeating. People who eat mindfully and slowly allow their bodies the time necessary to communicate satiety.

Accepting the Value of Emotional Intelligence: Recognizing Emotional Triggers Beyond the physical plane, mindfulness penetrates the emotional terrain of eating. People acquire the ability to recognize emotional cues and discern between true hunger and the need to use food as a calming or coping mechanism.

Lowering Anxiety and Stress: Reducing stress is facilitated by eating with awareness. People can foster a relaxing and well-digestive eating environment by being mindful and in the moment during meals.

Developing a Positive Relationship with Food: Mindful eating encourages a constructive and accepting mindset toward food. This in turn establishes the groundwork for a long-lasting and harmonious connection with eating patterns.

Long-Term Weight Management: Practicing mindfulness in intuitive dieting is a lifelong skill rather than a quick remedy. It gives people the resources they need to manage their weight over time and gives them the ability to make wise decisions in a variety of life circumstances.

Essentially, intuitive eating requires a conscious approach that extends beyond the plate to encompass all facets of life. People can change their connection with food and foster a sense of contentment, balance, and a deeper comprehension of the complex interactions between the mind and body by practicing present-moment mindfulness. We uncover the possibility of enduring well-being and revolutionary transformation as we explore the practical application of mindfulness in the context of intuitive dieting.

CHAPTER TWO

PRINCIPLES OF INTUITIVE DIETING

2.1 Intentional Eating

The foundation of intuitive dieting is mindful eating, which turns eating into a purposeful and fulfilling activity. Mindful eating creates a strong bond between people and the food they eat by activating the senses and developing present-moment awareness.

Essential Ideas for Mindful Eating

Savoring Every Bite: People who eat mindfully are encouraged to take their time and enjoy every meal. Meals can be more satisfying if one is aware of the flavors, textures, and scents of the food.

Eating with Intention: Mindful eating entails making a deliberate decision to feed the body rather than consuming meals on autopilot. It challenges people to consider their motivations for eating and determine if they are in line with emotional cues or bodily hunger.

How to Practice Mindful Eating in Real Life

Put an End to Distractions: Remove distractions from the dining area, such as television and technological devices. This makes it possible to engage with food in a concentrated and focused way.

Chewing Carefully: Eating mindfully entails giving each bite careful chewing. This helps people digest their meals better and lets them completely enjoy the flavors and textures of it.

Recognizing Cues of Hunger: Eating mindfully enables people to become aware of their bodies' hunger signals. This entails identifying the outward manifestations of hunger, such as a growling stomach or a feeling of emptiness.

Respecting Fullness: Honoring fullness is an equally significant behavior. Because they are aware of the small cues that signify fullness, mindful eaters can stop eating when they are content.

Beyond the Plate

Contemplative Meal Preparation: Incorporate mindfulness into meal preparation by taking dietary requirements and preferences into account. This guarantees that meals complement personal objectives and ideals.

Gratitude for Nourishment: Work on being appreciative of the food that is on your plate. Appreciating the work that went into creating and preparing the food is part of mindful eating.

Advantages of intentional eating

Weight management: By encouraging a more instinctive response to hunger and fullness cues and minimizing overeating, mindful eating has been associated with improved weight management.

Better Digestion: Mindful eating promotes optimal digestion and nutrient absorption by having people chew their food well and eat at a reasonable pace.

Enhanced Well-Being: Mindful eating promotes mental and emotional well-being in addition to physical health. Stress, worry, and emotional eating habits can all be lessened by it.

Mindful eating is a beacon that leads people into a closer relationship with their bodies and the food they offer in the intuitive dieting journey. We discover a revolutionary approach to not only what we eat but also how we interact with the act of eating as we investigate the real-world uses of mindful eating.

2.2 Positive Food Choices

Making healthy food choices that support one's mental and physical well-being is at the heart of the intuitive dieting philosophy. This feature encourages people to approach food with a sense of balance, mindfulness, and a true understanding of their own nutritional needs, as opposed to relying on strict dietary regulations. Below are some guiding concepts for making healthful food choices.

Density of nutrients: Give foods high in vital nutrients—like vitamins, minerals, and antioxidants—priority. These nutrient-dense options support general well-being and vigor.

Variety and Balance: To guarantee a well-balanced nutrient intake, embrace a wide variety of foods. Lean meats, whole grains, fruits, veggies, and healthy fats can all supply the body with a wide range of vital nutrients.

Paying Respect to Yourself: Embracing Your Needs: Intuitive dieting acknowledges that cravings are normal and could be a sign of dietary deficiencies. To foster a better connection with food, think about finding balanced ways to satiate cravings rather than fighting them.

Recognizing Sensitivities: Keep an eye on how your body reacts to certain foods. If some foods cause you discomfort or adverse reactions, think about making changes to your diet to support healthy digestion.

Continued Mindful Eating: Expand the mindful eating tenets to include food choosing. When making decisions, be mindful of the food's nutritional content and how it will affect your general health.

Moderation Is Key: Intuitive dieting places more emphasis on moderation than restriction. Instead of designating certain foods as "off-limits," adopt a balanced perspective and enjoy pleasures in moderation.

Developing Long-Term Habits: When it comes to intuitive dieting, making good food choices is more about developing long-lasting habits than it is about finding quick remedies. This strategy promotes long-term well-being and a positive connection with eating.

Tailoring Decisions to Your Lifestyle: Understand that each person has different nutritional requirements. Make dietary decisions based on your preferences, lifestyle, and health objectives to promote a sustainable and individualized eating style.

Creating a Good Connection with Food

Conscientious Consumption: Indulge in decadent foods with awareness and relish every second guilt-free. This strategy discourages the formation of negative attitudes toward particular meals and encourages a healthy relationship with treats.

Honoring nourishing: Consider food to be energy and a source of nourishment. Recognize the various ways that food supports your health and energy, and cultivate a positive outlook on eating.

A comprehensive approach to nutrition is created by combining mindful eating with positive food choices, which form the basis of intuitive dieting. Adopting a sustainable, personalized, and balanced approach to eating sets people on a path that goes beyond weight control and fosters a fulfilling and good connection with the food that their bodies are given.

2.3 Rejecting Diet Mentality

The rejection of the standard diet concept is a key component of intuitive dieting. This strategy encourages a mindset centered on self-compassion, balance, and long-term well-being by enabling people to break away from destructive dieting cycles rather than following rigid rules and outside norms.

Strict Rules: Conventional diets frequently impose rigid rules and limits, classifying foods as "good" or "bad." This is an example of understanding the diet mentality. This way of thinking can result in bad relationships with food as well as feelings of guilt and shame.

Short-Term Focus: Diets usually emphasize quick weight loss but do not provide a long-term, sustainable plan. This short-term concentration can lead to the yo-yo dieting cycle, in which people stop restrictive eating practices and then gain weight again.

Fundamentals of Resisting the Diet Mentality

Adopting Intuitive Eating: Intuitive dieting pushes people to adopt intuitive eating and trust their bodies. This entails paying attention to inner signals, respecting feelings of hunger and fullness, and selecting foods following personal needs.

Cultivating Self-Compassion: Developing self-compassion is a necessary step in rejecting the diet mindset. Individuals learn to be kind and empathetic to themselves instead of punishing themselves for imagined food transgressions.

Building a Positive Connection with Food

No Foods That Are "Bad" or "Good": Labeling foods as intrinsically good or harmful is a dichotomy that is challenged by intuitive dieting. A balanced diet can include any food, and the emphasis moves from restriction to focused enjoyment.

Breaking the Cycle of Guilt: People are urged to overcome the guilt they feel when they eat. A healthier connection with food is facilitated by realizing that occasional excesses are a normal part of life.

Tailoring Methods: Adopting a non-diet mindset entails realizing that there is no one-size-fits-all solution. People are free to personalize how they eat by taking into account lifestyle circumstances, cultural influences, and personal preferences.

Changing with Needs: Intuitive dieting acknowledges the dynamic nature of dietary requirements. Individuals' nutritional needs may vary as they get older, have various lifestyles, or deal with different health issues; eating habits should adjust to reflect these changes.

Encouraging Mental Health

Emphasis on Non-Scale milestones: When dieting intuitively, the emphasis is shifted from the scale's number to non-scale successes. Celebrating gains in vitality, happiness, and general health cultivates optimism.

Body Positivity: Developing body positivity is a necessary part of rejecting the diet mentality. A comprehensive and optimistic approach to well-being must include accepting and valuing one's body for its skills and distinctiveness.

Rejecting the diet mentality is a revolutionary step in the context of intuitive dieting toward creating a long-lasting and healthy relationship with food. Through the adoption of intuitive eating, self-compassion, and an emphasis on long-term health, people create pathways for a well-rounded and rewarding path to well-being.

CHAPTER THREE

INCORPORATING PHYSICAL ACTIVITY

3.1 Choosing Enjoyable Activities

Incorporating physical activity as a positive and joyful part of a healthy lifestyle is integral to the idea of intuitive dieting. Through the substitution of enjoyable activities for inflexible workout routines, people can develop a positive and long-lasting relationship with fitness and improve their general state of health.

Regaining Happiness Through Movement

Customized Exercise: Those who practice intuitive dieting are encouraged to experiment and find authentically enjoyable physical pursuits. The key is figuring out what personally resonates, whether that's dancing, hiking, swimming, or yoga.

Non-Traditional Exercise: Discover non-traditional ways to work out outside of the typical gym environment. Outside of the 'regimented' aspect of traditional workouts, leisure sports, gardening, and pet play all contribute to overall physical fitness.

Paying Attention to Your Body: Assessing Your Energy Levels Exercise is included in intuitive dieting since it encourages you to pay attention to your body's energy levels. Select pursuits that correspond with your energy level on any given day, understanding that exercise should feel energizing rather than draining.

Accepting Rest Days: The knowledge of rest is included in the intuitive exercise. Understand the value of taking days off to let your body heal and avoid burnout, which will help you maintain a sustainable and well-balanced exercise regimen.

Exercises for Mindful Movement

Tai Chi and Yoga: Include exercises for mindful movement such as tai chi or yoga. These activities support intuitive dieting's holistic tenets by improving mental clarity and relaxation in addition to physical health.

Explore contemplative walking as a type of physical activity. This is taking a leisure stroll, living in the present, and bringing mindfulness to the activity itself.

Creating an Active Lifestyle

Daily Movement: Replace your focus on regimented exercise with daily movement. This can entail doing things like walking during breaks, using the stairs, or participating in activities that naturally incorporate physical activity into daily life.

Social Activities: Take part in sports groups, group workshops, or outdoor activities with friends to combine socializing with fitness. This fosters social ties in addition to improving physical health.

Honoring Personal Development

Non-Competitive Method: The focus of the intuitive exercise is on a non-competitive methodology. Celebrate your personal improvement and the joy of activity instead of concentrating on performance measures.

Setting Achievable Goals: Include attainable exercise goals in your regimen. Your personal tastes should guide the creation of these goals so that you can feel motivated and accomplished without feeling overly pressured.

Selecting pleasurable activities is essential to building a healthy relationship with physical fitness in the context of intuitive dieting. By adopting a joyful movement, that fits personal preferences, and enhances overall well-being, people can develop a gratifying and long-lasting attitude to exercise that supports the holistic ideas of intuitive living.

3.2 Paying Attention to Your Body While Working Out

This method promotes a thoughtful and responsive attitude to physical activity by encouraging people to tune into their bodies' signals instead of following strict workout regimens.

Sensing Physical Feelings and Identifying

Comfort and Discomfort During workouts: Intuitive exercise requires being aware of your body's sensations. To ensure a safe and successful workout, learn to distinguish between the pain that indicates possible danger and the discomfort that comes with pushing boundaries.

Breath Awareness: During exercise, use your breathing as a guide. Pay attention to how you breathe and ensure it corresponds with how hard the exercise is. Regular, deep breathing improves general health and endurance.

Changing Intensity in Response to Energy Levels

Check-Ins on Energy: Check your energy levels frequently before, during, and after physical activity. Adapt the intensity of your exercise to your level of fitness, keeping in mind that some days may require more strenuous activity, and others may benefit from a softer regimen.

Accepting Variability: Exercise based on intuition recognizes that energy levels change. Accept variation in your exercise regimen, enabling yourself to adjust the level of intensity, length, and kind of activity according to what your body requires on any given day.

Considering Rest and Recuperation

Hearing Weariness: Keep an eye out for symptoms of fatigue and refrain from exerting oneself to the point of weariness. Honoring your body's desire for recuperation and realizing that rest is an essential part of a well-rounded fitness regimen are two aspects of intuitive exercise.

Including Active Recovery: Make active recovery days a part of your schedule by doing mild exercises like yoga, stretching, or walking. This promotes flexibility, circulation, and general healing without over-stressing the body.

Techniques for Mindful Movement

Body-Scan Meditation: To increase awareness of bodily sensations, practice body-scan meditation both before and after exercise. By fostering a better knowledge of your body's reactions to movement, this mindfulness method can help you establish connections with various parts of your body.

Stretching Intuitively: Instead of following a set of stretching schedules, concentrate on tense regions and move your body in ways that are comfortable and release tension.

Honoring Successes, both Large and Small

Non-Comparative Advancement Exercise based on intuition emphasizes individual growth more than outside standards. Celebrate your accomplishments instead of comparing yourself to others, whether they involve increased flexibility, endurance, or general well-being.

Creating Personal Objectives: Based on your unique experience, set attainable and customized exercise objectives. These objectives ought to be in line with your preferences and support an enjoyable and empowering workout.

A tenet of intuitive dieting is to listen to your body when exercising to foster a positive and balanced connection with physical activity. You may design a workout regimen that not only promotes your health but also adheres to the holistic ideas of intuitive living by tuning in to your body's signals, modifying intensity according to your energy levels, and adopting a mindful attitude to movement.

CHAPTER FOUR

MANAGING EMOTIONAL EATING

4.1 Recognizing Emotional Stressors

The process of identifying the particular circumstances, occurrences, or stimuli that cause people to experience emotions is known as emotional trigger identification. Since every individual has unique experiences, sensitivity levels, and traumatic histories that influence their emotional reactions, emotional triggers can fluctuate greatly from person to person. The following actions and things to think about can help you discover emotional triggers:

Self-knowledge: Urge people to consider their feelings and to be self-aware. Recognizing one's emotional responses is an essential first step in locating triggers. To keep track of your feelings and the situations that surround them, keep a notebook. Finding patterns and recurrent triggers can be aided by this.

Identify patterns: Examine emotional reactions for recurring patterns. Situations may be triggers if they frequently cause intense emotional reactions in you. Keep an eye on the length and intensity of emotional reactions. Emotions that are heightened by triggers frequently persist longer than usual.

Past experiences: Look into traumatic events and past experiences that might have contributed to emotional triggers. Emotions might be influenced by childhood experiences, past relationships, or important life events. Determine whether there are any unanswered questions or residual feelings from the past that may come up again in specific circumstances. Open communication should be fostered with others. Talking with loved ones, friends, or a therapist about feelings and triggers might yield insightful information. It's important to be open to comments from others regarding observed emotional reactions since they might see trends that people themselves might miss.

Observation and mindfulness: Develop mindfulness to increase your awareness of the here and now as well as your emotional condition. Triggers can be found in real-time with the use of mindful observation. Stay rooted in the here and now by practicing mindfulness exercises like deep breathing, meditation, or body scans. You can also notice your emotions without reacting right away.

Common triggers: Recognize the typical emotional triggers that you experience, including stress, rejection, criticism, loss, and change. These are common triggers that have varying effects on individuals. Recognize that for certain people, particular words, behaviors, or settings can also operate as triggers. People can learn more about their emotional triggers and create effective coping mechanisms by actively participating in self-reflection, asking for feedback from others, and being aware of their emotional reactions.

4.2 Creating Well-Being Coping Strategies

It is essential to establish good coping strategies to handle stress, overcome obstacles, and preserve emotional stability. The following are some practical methods for creating and using constructive coping mechanisms:

Self-awareness: Recognize when you are stressed, nervous, or overwhelmed by your feelings. Determine which certain triggers cause unfavorable feelings and take proactive measures to address them.

Meditation and mindfulness: To remain calm and present, engage in mindfulness practices like deep breathing exercises and meditation. A more impartial viewpoint and the ability to interrupt the loop of unfavorable ideas can both be fostered by mindfulness.

Exercise: Getting regular exercise helps alleviate tension and increases endorphins, which are endogenous hormones that naturally elevate mood. Getting regular exercise can help lower stress and enhance mental health in general.

Healthy Lifestyle Options: Give regular sleep, hydration, and a balanced diet priority. These elements have a big influence on how you feel and how well you can handle stress. Steer clear of excessive amounts of alcohol, coffee, and other chemicals that might exacerbate anxiety and tension.

Social Support: Preserve close relationships with loved ones, friends, and support networks. Communicate your feelings and views to those you can trust. Speaking with people at trying times can offer a variety of viewpoints and emotional support.

Time management: To efficiently manage your time, arrange and rank your tasks. Split more difficult jobs into smaller, more achievable portions. Stress and feelings of overload can be lessened by setting reasonable deadlines and goals. Effective problem-solving techniques should be developed in order to approach obstacles positively. Consider possible answers and take action to put them into practice rather than concentrating just on the issue at hand.

CHAPTER FIVE

BODY POSITIVITY AND ACCEPTANCE

5.1 Promoting a Healthful Self-Image

Promoting a healthy body image is crucial for mental and general well-being. The following are some methods for encouraging a positive body image:

Develop self-compassion by treating oneself with kindness and compassion: Show yourself the same consideration that you would a friend. Positive and uplifting statements should take the place of negative self-talk and be challenged.

Put Function First: Pay more attention to what your body is capable of doing rather than how it looks. Honor its tenacity, fortitude, and the pursuits it permits you to undertake. Instead of evaluating your body purely based on appearance, embrace its capabilities.

Increase Your Exposure to Diverse Media: Watch and listen to media that highlights many body types and encourages people of all shapes, sizes, and looks. Restrict your exposure to media that damages body image and upholds unattainable beauty ideals.

Be in the Company of Positive People: Create a welcoming environment for yourself by associating with those who uphold a positive view of oneself and one's body. Talk about skills, capabilities, and accomplishments instead of looks in your conversations.

Establish Achievable and Realistic Objectives: Make sure your health and wellness objectives are centered on your total well-being rather than a certain body type or weight. Celebrate and acknowledge your progress instead of focusing on perfection.

Contest Beauty Ideals: Contest the conventions and expectations of beauty in society, understanding that there is no one "ideal" body type for beauty, there are many different types of it. Accept differences and value the distinctive qualities of various bodies.

Constructive affirmations: Work constructive affirmations into your everyday routine. Remind yourself that you are valuable in ways that go beyond looks. Recite affirmations that support acceptance and self-love.

Take Part in Things You Love: Do things that make you happy and fulfilled, and don't worry about how you look while you're doing them. Seek out pursuits that feed your body and mind and enhance your overall sense of well-being.

Develop Gratitude: Develop an appreciation for your body and all that it does. Recognize and value the complex systems that allow you to lead a happy life. Consistently acknowledge the good things in your body.

Educate Yourself: Get knowledge on how the media affects body image and the impracticality of many beauty standards. You can change your perspective by realizing that much of what is portrayed as "ideal" is frequently contrived and unreachable.

Recall that developing a good relationship with yourself is a necessary step in maintaining a positive body image. Remain calm, treat yourself with kindness, and acknowledge the special qualities and powers of your body.

5.2 Honoring Achievements That Aren't Scale

Promoting a healthy and optimistic mindset is crucial, especially when it comes to fitness and overall well-being, and celebrating non-scale wins is one way to do this. Non-scale victories (NSVs) are accomplishments and constructive adjustments that surpass a scale point. Observe these methods for acknowledging non-scale successes:

Track Your Progress Beyond Weight: Monitor your fitness and health in addition to your weight loss. Enhancements in strength, stamina, flexibility, or general energy levels could fall under this category.

Fit and Comfort of Clothes: Rejoice when formerly tight clothing fits more easily or you can wear it again. Appreciate the good changes in the shape and composition of your body and concentrate on how you feel about yourself in your clothes.

Enhanced Energy: Observe any increases in your level of energy. It is a non-scale triumph if you experience an increase in energy, alertness, and focus. An increase in energy is frequently a sign of healthy lifestyle modifications and general well-being.

Better Habits: Celebrate and acknowledge the adoption of better habits, including choosing wholesome foods, drinking enough of water, or exercising frequently. Acknowledge the benefits these practices bring to your general well-being and energy.

Mental and Emotional Well-Being: Honor advancements in your emotional and mental health. Think of these non-scale successes if you feel less stressed, happier, or more confident. Improvements in mental health are important markers of general well-being.

Regularity in Habits: Rather than concentrating just on immediate results, acknowledge the regularity in your healthy routines. Persistently good behavior is typically the key to long-term success. Acknowledge the work you do to keep your lifestyle healthy.

Fitness Accomplishments: Be proud of your accomplishments in terms of fitness, such as reaching a new workout level, lifting more weights, or jogging a specific distance. Celebrate your accomplishments and increased level of fitness.

Body Measurements: Monitor variations in your waist, hips, and thighs. Positive shifts in these directions may have greater significance than shifts in the scale. To track development over time, use a tape measure.

Higher Quality Sleep: Honor gains in both the quantity and quality of your slumber. Requiring enough sleep has a favorable effect on many areas of your life and is necessary for general health. Congratulate yourself for making progress in your positive self-talk and thinking. It's a huge non-scale win if you're evolving toward a more positive and self-affirming mindset about your body.

Social Support and Community: Celebrate the connections you've built with others who share similar health and fitness goals. Supportive social networks contribute to a positive and motivating environment. Remember, the journey to improved health is multifaceted, and the scale is just one measure of progress. By acknowledging and celebrating non-scale victories, you shift the focus from a number to the positive changes and improvements in various aspects of your life and well-being.

Journaling: Write down your ideas and feelings in a journal. Writing can be a therapeutic means of gaining an understanding of your experiences and processing feelings. Track patterns, pinpoint triggers, and keep tabs on your coping development by keeping a journal.

Relaxation Methods: To relieve stress, experiment with methods like progressive muscle relaxation, guided visualization, or aromatherapy. Seek out peaceful activities and include them in your daily schedule.

Hobbies and Leisure Activities: Take part in enjoyable and soothing activities. Interests and recreational activities can enhance general well-being and serve as a constructive diversion.

Keep in mind that creating effective coping methods takes time and that different people require various approaches. Try out different methods to see which one suits you the best, and be kind to yourself while you develop a toolkit of useful coping mechanisms.

CHAPTER SIX

REGULAR CHECK-INS AND ADJUSTMENTS

6.1 Evaluating the Effect of Foods

Evaluating the effects of food on your general health, overall well-being, and individual health goals is part of assessing the impact of food. This procedure takes into account factors more than just calorie counting, such as nutritional value, possible allergies, and personal food reactions. When evaluating the effects of foods, take into account the following important factors: Foods should be evaluated for their nutritional content, taking into account both macronutrients (proteins, fats, and carbohydrates) and micronutrients (vitamins and minerals). To guarantee a well-rounded and balanced diet, select a range of nutrient-dense foods.

Personal Dietary Requirements: Take into account your unique dietary requirements, which can change depending on your age, gender, degree of exercise, and health. Tailor your diet to fulfill certain dietary needs and correct any inadequacies.

Food Allergies and Sensitivities: Recognize any dietary sensitivities or allergies you may have. Shellfish, dairy, nuts, and gluten are common allergies. If you are aware of any allergies or sensitivities, carefully read food labels and select alternatives.

Glycemic Index and Blood Sugar Effect: Recognize food's glycemic index (GI), particularly if you're watching your blood sugar levels or worry about insulin resistance. To assist in stabilizing blood sugar levels; choose foods with lower GI values.

Assess how drinks affect your level of hydration: Hydration is important for general health and sugar-filled beverages and high caffeine intake can dehydrate people. Ensure you drink sufficient water all through the day to sustain appropriate hydration.

Timing and Frequency of Meals: Take into account the times and dates of your meals. While some people might benefit from larger, less frequent meals, others might prefer smaller, more regular meals. Consider how the timing and frequency of your meals affect your digestion, energy levels, and general health.

Whole foods and processed foods: In general, whole foods with less processing, such as fruits, vegetables, and lean proteins, are higher in nutrients. Eat less highly processed meals that contain unnatural additives, bad fats, and added sugars.

Portion Sizes: To prevent overindulging, pay attention to portion sizes. To aid with portion control, think about using smaller dishes and pay attention to signals of hunger and fullness. For both weight control and general health, portion control is essential.

Cultural and Individual Preferences: When evaluating the effects of foods, take into account cultural and individual preferences. A fulfilling and long-lasting diet can be achieved by consuming a range of foods that suit your own preferences and cultural background.

Digestive Health: Be mindful of how certain foods affect the condition of your digestive system. Certain meals, including dairy or high-fiber diets, may cause pain or digestive problems for certain people. Try several diets to find foods that support the best possible digestion. Dietary decisions can be improved and adjusted when you periodically reevaluate how foods affect your health. Remember that everyone reacts differently to different foods, so it's important to listen to your body and make decisions that suit your own requirements and objectives. For individualized advice, think about speaking with a registered dietitian or other healthcare provider if you have any particular health issues or food limitations.

6.2 Modifying Consumption Patterns

Changing one's eating habits is a dynamic process that calls for self-awareness as well as a determination to make better decisions. Here are some tips for improving your eating habits, regardless of whether your goals are to lose weight, enhance your nutrition, or take care of a particular health issue:

Establish Achievable and Realistic Goals: Establish measurable objectives for your eating habits. To make development more achievable, break down bigger objectives into smaller, more doable steps. Track What You Eat, When You Eat It, and How You Feel During and After Meals by Keeping a Food Journal. Finding trends and potential improvement areas can be aided by this.

Recognize Portion Sizes: To prevent overindulging, familiarize yourself with appropriate serving sizes. To determine the right serving sizes, use measurement devices or visual cues.

Increased Consumption of Fruits and Vegetables: Make an effort to incorporate a range of fruits and vegetables into your meals. These foods support general health since they are high in fiber, antioxidants, vitamins, and minerals.

Harmonize Macronutrients: Try to consume lipids, proteins, and carbohydrates in a balanced manner. For long-lasting energy, combine whole grains, lean meats, and healthy fats in your meals.

Select Whole Foods: Give preference to minimally processed, whole foods over those that have undergone extensive processing. Whole foods are often healthier options since they retain more of their nutrients.

Sustain Hydration: All through the day, drink an adequate amount of water. Feelings of hunger can occasionally be mistaken for dehydration.

Limit Processed Foods and Added Sugars: Cut back on the amount of foods and drinks that include processed components and added sugars. Look for hidden sugars on food labels and choose full, nutrient-dense foods instead.

Plan and Prepare Meals: To prevent relying on unhealthy, convenient options, plan your meals. You have control over the ingredients and portion quantities when you cook at home.

Practice Moderation: Adopt a moderate mindset as opposed to one of severe restrictions. Treat yourself periodically, but don't overindulge to avoid feeling constrained.

Pay Attention to Your Body: Monitor your body signals when it is starving or full. Rather than consuming everything on your plate, eat when you're hungry and stop when you're full.

Seek Help: Discuss your objectives with loved ones, close friends, or a support group. Support networks can offer drive, accountability, and encouragement.

Gradual Adjustments: Make adjustments bit by bit. More often than not, small, sustainable changes turn into long-lasting habits as opposed to large, fast fixes. Adopting healthier eating habits over the long run is considerably aided by consistency and a good mentality.

CHAPTER SEVEN

PROFESSIONAL GUIDANCE

7.1 Speak with a Certified Dietitian

Addressing a variety of health and nutrition-related issues can benefit from speaking with a Registered Dietitian (RD). Having completed specialized study and training in nutrition, registered dietitians are skilled professionals who frequently possess a degree in dietetics or a closely related discipline.

Advantages and justifications for speaking with an RD

Personalized Nutrition Plans: To develop a personalized nutrition plan, registered dietitians can evaluate your unique food preferences, lifestyle, and health concerns. A registered dietitian (RD) can customize advice to meet your specific needs, whether you're trying to manage a medical condition, reduce weight, or improve your general well-being.

Evidence-Based Guidance: RDs rely on empirical data to support their recommendations. They can offer knowledge that is dependable and trustworthy since they keep up with the most recent developments in nutrition research. This is especially crucial in a time when there is a lot of false information on diet.

Medical Nutrition Therapy: Registered Dietitians (RDs) can offer medical nutrition therapy to people with certain medical illnesses, such as diabetes, cardiovascular disease, or gastrointestinal issues. In collaboration with other medical specialists, this entails adopting nutrition treatments to control or treat certain health issues.

Weight Management: An RD can assist you in creating a sustainable and well-balanced eating plan if your goal is to reach and stay at a healthy weight. They can offer advice on meal planning, portion management, and behavior modification techniques.

Allergies and Intolerances: An RD can help you create a well-balanced diet while avoiding particular allergens if you have any food allergies or intolerances. They can guarantee that, even with dietary restrictions, you still get all the nutrients you need.

Sports Nutrition: Consulting with a registered dietitian (RD) can help athletes maximize their nutritional intake for optimal performance. This covers tips on fueling before, during, and following exercise in addition to recovery and hydration techniques.

Lifestyle Modifications: It can be difficult to alter dietary habits. You can make practical and long-lasting dietary adjustments with the assistance of an RD.

Maintenance of Long-Term Health: RDs prioritize maintaining long-term well-being and health. They can assist you in forming routines that support a healthy lifestyle and guard against any health problems.

You may usually locate a registered dietitian through medical facilities, community health centers, private practices, or internet resources if you're thinking about scheduling a consultation. Remember that although other nutritionists can offer helpful advice, the label "Registered Dietitian" is protected and denotes a specific degree of training and certification. Make sure the nutritionist you select has the necessary certifications.

7.2 Seeking Assistance for Mental Health

Starting a weight loss journey can have an impact on one's physical and mental well-being. It's crucial to approach weight loss with an emphasis on general well-being, and getting help for your mental health is a key part of this process.

Here are some recommendations

Treatment or Counseling: If you're having difficulty in controlling your weight, eating disorders, or anxiety over body image, do well to seek advice from a therapist. They can support you in identifying and resolving any underlying emotional issues that are influencing your desire to lose weight.

Support Groups: Participating in an online or in-person support group helps foster a feeling of understanding and camaraderie. Making connections with people who are traveling comparable paths can provide encouragement, motivation, and common experiences.

Stress Management and Mindfulness: Use mindfulness practices to control your stress levels and emotional eating. You can increase your awareness of your feelings and responses by practicing mindfulness-based stress reduction, deep breathing exercises, and meditation.

Body Positivity and Self-Love: Develop a loving relationship with your body and yourself. This entails realizing that physical beauty is not the only factor in determining one's self-worth and accepting and appreciating your body at every stage of your journey.

Establish sensible objectives: Set attainable and reasonable weight loss objectives. Unreasonable expectations have a detrimental effect on mental health and can cause frustration. Reward yourself for little accomplishments and growth, and practice self-compassion.

Prioritize Health over Weight: Change your attention from merely reducing weight to enhancing your general health. Include routines that promote your health, such as eating a well-balanced diet, getting enough exercise, and getting enough sleep.

Seek advice from medical professionals: A certified dietitian or nutritionist should be a part of your team of healthcare specialists to help you lose weight in a way that is safe, sustainable, and customized for you.

Taking Consistent Stocks of Yourself: Check in with your feelings and mental health regularly. Keeping a journal can help you analyze your emotions, spot trends, and monitor your development.

Honor Non-Scale Victories: Give credit to accomplishments that go above and beyond the scale, including greater energy, a happier disposition, or improved levels of fitness.

Seek Assistance from Friends and Family: Discuss your objectives with understanding and encouraging friends and family members. Having a solid support network is crucial for maintaining mental health when trying to lose weight.

Recall that general health is closely related to mental health. Do not hesitate to get professional assistance if you are experiencing emotional difficulties or if your relationship with food starts to become difficult. A mental health expert can offer support, coping mechanisms, and direction specific to your needs and situation.

CHAPTER EIGHT

SUSTAINABLE INTUITIVE LIFESTYLE AND WELL-BEING

8.1: Adopting an Intuitive and Sustainable Lifestyle

Making deliberate decisions that are good for people and the environment is a necessary step toward living an intuitive and sustainable lifestyle. Intuition is essential to this process because it prompts people to follow their principles and pay attention to their inner guidance. An intuitive lifestyle encourages people to think about the social and environmental effects of their decisions rather than following strict restrictions. This could be choosing organic and locally sourced goods, adopting a more minimalist lifestyle, and minimizing waste via thoughtful consumption. By developing a stronger sense of connection with the environment and a sense of responsibility for the health of the earth, people can enhance their intuition.

Steps in adopting an intuitive and sustainable lifestyle

A thoughtful set of actions that add up to a more balanced and environmentally responsible way of life is required to embrace an intuitive and sustainable existence. Increasing awareness and educating oneself on how one's decisions affect the environment is one of the first steps in the process. Knowing how items are made, the effects of excessive consumption, and the advantages of going with sustainable options are all part of this. Decisions that are in line with sustainability principles can only be made with the support of knowledge.

The next stage after gaining awareness is to evaluate and reduce one's ecological footprint. This entails assessing everyday routines, including energy use, waste production, and transportation, and pinpointing areas in need of improvement. Making minor adjustments like taking public transit, using less water and electricity, and recycling can add up to have a big positive influence. Here, the emphasis is on making small changes at first and realizing that they add up to a more sustainable way of living.

Adopting an intuitive lifestyle also requires embracing a deliberate and thoughtful approach to eating. This means considering whether purchases are really necessary, choosing quality over quantity, and endorsing products that are ethical and environmentally sustainable. You can further lessen your product's impact on the environment by selecting items with minimum packaging and those made of recycled or renewable materials. Additionally, a minimalist mindset can aid in life de-cluttering, encouraging a deeper relationship with belongings and lowering consumption levels.

A natural and intuitive lifestyle must have a strong connection to the natural world. A greater awareness and respect for the environment are fostered by spending time outside, whether it is for hiking, gardening, or just taking in the scenery. A stronger dedication to environmental protection is frequently the result of this link. Furthermore, a holistic and sustainable lifestyle is facilitated by implementing sustainable practices in personal health, such as plant-based diets, eco-friendly workout regimens, and mindfulness exercises that prioritize mental well-being.

Essentially, living a sustainable and intuitive lifestyle is an ongoing process characterized by deliberate decisions and a dedication to making beneficial changes. Every action, no matter how tiny, makes a difference in the overall endeavor to live sustainably and to encourage a more balanced and meaningful life. As people advance on this road, they contribute significantly to building a more resilient and sustainable future for the world in addition to improving their own well-being.

8.2: Persisting in the Pursuit of Greater Well-Being

Persistence is essential to the intuitive dieting journey in order to achieve better health. By focusing on a conscious and innate relationship with one's body and its dietary demands, intuitive dieting goes beyond conventional methods. It necessitates an unwavering dedication to paying attention to the body's signals and cues, cultivating a profound comprehension of hunger, satisfaction, and general well-being. There may be obstacles along the road on the intuitive dieting route to better health and vitality. But what distinguishes the tenacious person on this life-changing adventure is their ability to bounce back from setbacks and adjust. When one continues to foster a positive relationship with food and body, the benefits become apparent in better mental and physical health as well as a long-term nutrition plan that suits each person's needs. The secret to achieving a balanced and satisfying existence, where the quest for improved well-being becomes a lifetime commitment steered by self-awareness and thoughtful decisions, is, in essence, perseverance in intuitive dieting.

Steps in **persisting in the pursuit of greater well-being**

Maintaining a diet and weight loss regimen as a means of achieving better health requires a more comprehensive strategy than band-aid solutions. Setting attainable and realistic goals is the first step. Instead of concentrating only on a goal weight, people can think about more general health goals like more energy, better mood, and better physical fitness. Setting realistic goals contributes to the development of an inspiring and long-lasting foundation for success.

Creating a solid support network is essential to keeping the momentum going in the direction of improved well-being. Establishing a community of like-minded people or sharing your objectives with friends and family can help you stay accountable and gain insightful feedback. A sense of community is fostered by having a support system, which makes the journey less lonely and more pleasurable. Honoring successes—no matter how minor—becomes a communal event that strengthens dedication.

Keeping up the good work on the road to increased well-being also requires incorporating mindful eating habits. This entails being aware of signals of hunger and fullness, enjoying every meal, and selecting foods with awareness. A better relationship with food is facilitated by mindful eating, which also helps to curb impulsive or emotional eating. To improve one's overall path toward well-being, one should cultivate an awareness of one's nutritional demands and enjoy a range of nourishing foods.

A healthy weight requires regular physical exercise to be attained and maintained. People might engage in activities they truly enjoy instead of seeing fitness as a chore. Finding pleasurable ways to exercise increases the likelihood that it will become a regular part of one's routine, whether that activity is hiking, dancing, cycling, or practicing yoga. A sustainable approach to fitness is ensured by establishing reasonable workout goals and escalating intensity gradually.

Along the path to well-being, it's critical to adopt an optimistic outlook and exercise patience. It takes time to lose weight and modify one's lifestyle, and obstacles are a normal part of the journey. Rather than considering setbacks as failures, people can regard them as chances to grow and modify their strategy.

Recognizing accomplishments boosts motivation and solidifies the will to lead a healthier lifestyle.

A vital part of continuing the quest for improved health is educating oneself about nutrition and implementing a sustainable, well-balanced diet. This means knowing what meals are good for you, making wise decisions, and staying away from diets that are too severe or trendy. Overall health is supported and feelings of deprivation are avoided with a varied and well-rounded diet rich in nutrient-dense foods.

Last but not least, consulting a professional can offer insightful advice and customized plans for boosting well-being. Advice based on personal requirements and objectives can be customized by speaking with a registered dietitian, nutritionist, or fitness specialist. The chosen strategy is guaranteed to be safe, successful, and in line with long-term well-being goals when professional guidance is obtained.

In summary, pursuing greater well-being through dieting and weight loss requires setting realistic goals, creating a network of support, practicing mindful eating, getting physical exercise that you enjoy, keeping a positive outlook, learning about nutrition, and consulting a professional. People can develop enduring habits that improve their general health and well-being by taking a holistic and sustainable approach.

CHAPTER NINE

CONCLUSION

By way of conclusion, "Intuitive Dieting and Weight Loss" invites readers on a transformative journey toward a healthier relationship with food, their bodies, and ultimately, themselves. Through the exploration of intuitive eating principles, mindfulness practices, and the integration of mental health support, this book seeks to redefine the conventional narrative surrounding weight loss. It emphasizes the importance of self-compassion, realistic goal-setting, and the acknowledgment of non-scale victories as crucial components of a holistic approach to well-being.

Readers are encouraged to embrace a more intuitive, sustainable approach to weight control as they work through the book's pages and toss aside strict dieting guidelines. Through the cultivation of mindfulness, the promotion of a positive body image, and the pursuit of external and internal support, people can undertake a journey that goes beyond simple physical change. The end objective isn't just a number on the scale; rather, it's a significant mental shift that results in enhanced self-love, better mental health, and a sustainable, lifetime commitment to general happiness and health.

With a balanced and intuitive approach to dieting and weight loss, may this book act as a guide, enabling readers to trust their bodies, make conscious decisions, and experience joy and contentment. In the end, pursuing well-being is a journey that never ends—one that leads to a more fulfilling, healthful life.

9 7 9 8 8 7 3 8 8 2 0 5 2